Union Calendar No. 7

113TH CONGRESS		REPORT
1st Session	" HOUSE OF REPRESENTATIVES !	113–11

"BILLIONS OF FEDERAL TAX DOLLARS MISSPENT ON NEW YORK'S MEDICAID PROGRAM"

REPORT

BY THE

COMMITTEE ON OVERSIGHT AND GOVERNMENT REFORM

MARCH 5, 2013.—Committed to the Committee of the Whole House on the State of the Union and ordered to be printed

———

U.S. GOVERNMENT PRINTING OFFICE

29–006   WASHINGTON : 2013

LETTER OF TRANSMITTAL

HOUSE OF REPRESENTATIVES,
COMMITTEE ON OVERSIGHT AND GOVERNMENT REFORM,
Washington, DC, March 5, 2013.

Hon. JOHN BOEHNER,
The Speaker, House of Representatives,
Washington, DC.

DEAR MR. SPEAKER: By direction of the Committee on Oversight and Government Reform, I submit herewith the Committee's report to the 113th Congress. This report was adopted by the Committee on February 13, 2013, in a meeting that was open to the public.

Sincerely,

DARRELL ISSA,
Chairman.

CONTENTS

	Page
Executive Summary	1
I. Introduction	3
II. New York's Medicaid Program is the Largest in the Country	5
III. Examples of Problems in New York's Medicaid Program	6
Lack of Controls and Misspending in New York's Personal Care Services Medicaid program [1]	
Overpayments to New York Developmental Centers	
Abuses of Medicaid Eligibility Rules in New York	
Excessive Salaries Paid to Executives of Medicaid-funded Organizations	
IV. Patient Abuse Within the Developmentally Disabled System in New York	
V. Past Health Care-related Corruption by Elected Officials	14
VI. Allegations of Problems with State Oversight of the Medicaid Program	16
VII. Reforms in the Last Two Years and Additional Concerns	17
VIII. Recommendations	23
IX. Conclusion	25
Appendix A	26
Appendix B	26
Appendix C	29
Committee Consideration; Statement of Oversight Findings and Recommendation of the Committee; Statement of General Performance Goals and Objectives	32

[1] For more information about Personal Care Services in New York and Dr. Feldman's testimony before the Committee, see the Committee Staff Report entitled Uncovering Waste, Fraud, and Abuse in the Medicaid Program, U S. House Committee on Oversight & Gov't Reform (April 25, 2012) [hereinafter Committee Staff Report].

Union Calendar No. 7

"BILLIONS OF FEDERAL TAX DOLLARS MISSPENT ON NEW YORK'S MEDICAID PROGRAM"

MARCH 5, 2013.—Committed to the Committee of the Whole House on the State of the Union and ordered to be printed

Mr. ISSA, from the Committee on Oversight and Government Reform, submitted the following

R E P O R T

EXECUTIVE SUMMARY

New York State's Medicaid program is the largest in the country. In fiscal year 2010, New York's $2,700 per resident Medicaid spending exceeded per capita Medicaid spending in the rest of the country by more than $1,500. When problems have been identified, the cost associated has often been large as well. Poor program oversight by both the State and federal Government has contributed to these problems.

This report discusses past findings of the Office of Inspector General (OIG) of the Department of Health and Human Services (HHS), investigative reporters, whistle-blowers and this Committee of waste, fraud, and abuse within New York's Medicaid program. It also discusses positive steps taken by Governor Andrew Cuomo to address many of those problems, highlights continuing concerns, and offers several recommendations aimed at protecting future tax dollars from being misspent. Several of the costly problems discussed in this report include:

• In 2010, the Poughkeepsie Journal reported that Medicaid was paying extremely high payment rates for residents in New York's State-operated developmental centers. The high payments resulted from a complicated methodology that was initially approved more than two decades ago by the Federal Government. This methodology resulted in daily payment rates exceeding $5,000 for each institutional resident by 2011. The Committee majority estimates that the Federal share of total payments going to the State through these facilities was approximately $15 billion in excess of a reasonable amount. The Centers for Medicare and Medicaid Services (CMS) believes that the developmental center payments exceeded Medicaid upper payment limits established by Congress. The excessive rates have remained in place for two-and-a-half years after the Federal Government began asking the State for information about the developmental center payment rates.

• Over the past decade, HHS OIG has uncovered ten instances in which New York State has improperly claimed at least $50 million in Federal Medicaid dollars. Moreover, in the past four years, the Federal Government has successfully sued New York for unlawful Medicaid expenditures twice, recovering more than $600 million.

• In 2009, a whistle-blower sued New York City for rampant inappropriate and fraudulent spending in Medicaid's Personal Care Services (PCS) program.

• The Committee has learned that Medicaid estate planning is a long-standing practice and significant problem across the nation and in New York State. The Committee has learned that relatively affluent people in New York artificially impoverish themselves in order to qualify for Medicaid and have taxpayers pick up the cost of their long-term care services and supports. At least in Suffolk County, New York, a relatively affluent part of the State, a legal technique called spousal refusal, which is essentially when one spouse abandons all financial care of a sick or disabled spouse and leaves him or her as a ward of the State, is widely used.

• The Committee has uncovered excessive salaries paid to executives of nonprofit institutions that are nearly completely financed by Medicaid. The Committee found that at least 15 of these executives received yearly compensation exceeding $500,000 and at least 100 others received yearly compensation exceeding $200,000.

• Over the past decade, many powerful elected members of New York's State legislature, including two recent State Senate majority leaders, have been convicted of fraud or corruption charges related to health care.

• Reforming Medicaid in New York faces several significant challenges. For one, many powerful special interest groups in New York benefit from the State's large Medicaid expenditures and lobby strongly against changes that would reform the State's program. Another challenge is the long-standing New York practice of increasing Medicaid as a way to leverage extra Federal money into the State.

At the beginning of his term, Governor Andrew Cuomo called New York's Medicaid program "bloated" and argued that it "must be reformed to help [New York] [S]tate begin to make ends meet." The Committee has also found that despite these obstacles, several program reforms are being orchestrated by the Cuomo Administration, including:

• The Cuomo Administration has enacted many new policies through a Medicaid Redesign program, including the first-in-the-nation Medicaid global cap, which places a budget constraint on the State's Medicaid spending. There is also evidence that the State has had some initial success with reducing waste, fraud, and abuse within New York City's PCS Medicaid program.

• Finally, after two decades of overpayments, New York and CMS are in the midst of negotiations to develop an appropriate rate and come to an appropriate amount for the Federal Government to recoup for past overpayments in excess of reasonable costs.

• Early last year, Governor Cuomo issued an executive order which limits executive compensation at Medicaid-financed institutions to less than $199,000.

While New York's actions over the past few years are a step in the right direction, it is clear to the Committee that there is more that New York and the Federal Government can do to make the State's Medicaid program more cost-effective. The Committee recommends six specific actions that should be taken immediately to reduce Medicaid waste, fraud, and abuse in New York's program and potentially save both Federal and New York State taxpayers significant amounts of money each year:

• CMS or a qualified government watchdog agency should conduct a complete and independent audit of New York's Medicaid program, including the work of New York State's Office of the Medicaid Inspector General;

• CMS should finalize an agreement with New York on a corrected payment methodology that ends the developmental center overpayments as soon as possible. CMS should pursue recovery of an appropriate portion of previous overpayments in excess of reasonable costs for Federal taxpayers;

• CMS' review of New York's Section 1115 waiver request, to allow the State to keep a portion of the savings its Medicaid reforms are projected to achieve should follow all applicable statutory requirements, particularly with respect to budget neutrality. CMS should also ensure that the baseline from which New York is calculating the savings does not include developmental center overpayments or other overpayments;

• New York's PCS program must only enroll individuals who meet the eligibility thresholds required by law;

• New York's legislature should ban "spousal refusal" and other abuses of Medicaid eligibility rules, as Governor Cuomo has proposed in each of his three budgets. New York must also aggressively pursue estate recovery against people who abuse Medicaid eligibility rules; and

• New York's legislature should codify Governor Cuomo's executive order limiting compensation of executives at organizations receiving nearly all their money from tax revenue. New York must also aggressively monitor and enforce these limits.

I. INTRODUCTION

In June 2011, nearly 53 million Americans were enrolled in Medicaid, a joint Federal-State program that finances health and long-term care services for a diverse group of individuals.[2] While Federal law currently mandates certain minimum coverage standards for state Medicaid programs, states can—and very often do—expand eligibility criteria and benefits beyond mandated thresholds. Adjusted for inflation, Medicaid spending has increased over 250 percent since 1990,[3] and government experts estimate that Med-

---

[2] Kaiser Commission on Medicaid Facts, Medicaid Enrollment: June 2011 Data Snapshot, available at: http://www.kff.org/medicaid/upload/8050-05.pdf.

[3] In 1990, national expenditures on Medicaid equaled $73.7 billion. (See National Health Expenditures, Levels and Annual Change, Table 3, Center for Medicaid and CHIP Services, avail-

Continued

icaid cost American taxpayers $440 billion in 2012.[4] The Federal Government reimburses state Medicaid spending, typically equal to half of Medicaid expenditures in states with the highest per capita income, and about 75 percent in states with the lowest per capita income.[5] In aggregate, the Federal Government typically reimburses about 57 percent of state Medicaid spending, and in New York the typical Federal reimbursement is 50 percent.[6]

To put the size of the program in context, annual Medicaid spending now exceeds Wal-Mart's worldwide annual revenue and is more than 50 percent larger than Greece's entire economy.[7] The Committee majority believes an uncapped Federal reimbursement makes this the program particularly susceptible to waste, fraud and abuse. As explained in an April 2012 Republican staff report:

> The policy of an open-ended federal reimbursement of state Medicaid spending significantly reduces the incentives for states to act as wise stewards of federal tax dollars. For example, in order to return $1,000 in fraudulent Medicaid funding for state purposes, a state with a 60% federal Medicaid reimbursement rate would have to identify and recover $2,500 of waste, fraud, and abuse in its program. Since 60% of the total recovery would have to be returned to the U.S. Treasury, the state would have to refund $1,500 of the $2,500 it recovered. Moreover, due to the open-ended federal Medicaid reimbursement, many states view Medicaid as an economic growth engine and therefore lack much interest in where the money is going. States would also have to increase resources to uncover the waste, fraud, and abuse. For these reasons, the federal Medicaid reimbursement demonstrates one of the core reasons the Medicaid program suffers from rampant waste, fraud, and abuse.[8]

Each Federal dollar misspent on Medicaid is one less dollar for the country to use for better health care for the poor, education, infrastructure, national defense, deficit reduction, or any other priority. One concern is that some politicians and policymakers view Medicaid not only as a program to assist low-income and disabled persons access health care and long-term care services, but also as a way to bring Federal dollars into the State.

The Committee discovered a decades-long problem in New York's Medicaid program, which is the subject of this Committee Report.

---

able at http://www.cms.gov/Research-Statistics-Data-and-Systems/Statistics-Trends-and-Reports/NationalHealthExpendData/Downloads/tables.pdf.) Adjusted for inflation, this would equal about $129.5 in 2012 dollars since the average annual consumer price index was 130.7 in 1990 and 229.594 in 2012. (*See* Consumer Price Index, Bureau of Labor Statistics, U.S. Dept. of Labor, available at ftp://ftp.bls.gov/pub/special.requests/cpi/cpiai.txt.)

[4] Spending and Enrollment Detail for CBO's February 2013 Baseline: Medicaid.

[5] Federal Financial Participation in State Assistance Expenditures; Federal Matching Shares for Medicaid, the Children's Health Insurance Program, and Aid to Needy, Aged, Blind or Disabled Persons for FY 2012, 75 Fed. Reg. 69082, 69083 (Nov. 9, 2010), available at http://aspe.hhs.gov/health/fmap12.shtml.

[6] The American Recovery and Reinvestment Act raised the average reimbursement rate for the U.S. States to nearly 70 percent for fiscal years 2009 through 2011. Between fiscal year 2008 and fiscal year 2009, the average State FMAP increased from 59.7% to 70.0%. Kaiser Family Foundation State Health Facts, Federal Medical Assistance Percentage (FMAP) for Medicaid and Multiplier, available at http://www.statehealthfacts.org/comparetable.jsp?ind=184&cat=4.

[7] According to the World Bank, Greece's Gross Domestic Product was slightly under $290 billion in 2011. *See* Greece, The World Bank, available at http://data.worldbank.org/country/greece.

[8] *See* Committee Staff Report, *supra* note 1.

II. NEW YORK'S MEDICAID PROGRAM IS THE LARGEST IN THE COUNTRY

New York's spending on Medicaid is the highest in the country by a considerable amount. Table 1 shows Medicaid per resident spending in Fiscal Year (FY) 2010 on the program's three main spending categories—acute care, long-term care, and disproportionate share hospitals (DSH) [9]—for California, New York, Pennsylvania, and the entire country. The numbers in parentheses show how many dollars New York spends per resident on Medicaid spending for every dollar spent per capita in each of the other three regions. As Table 1 shows, New York's per resident Medicaid spending is nearly double that of Pennsylvania and more than double that of California and the entire country. Appendix A contains a table that shows the Federal share of state Medicaid spending for FY 2010 on a per capita basis for all 50 States. Federal taxpayers contributed $1,657 toward New York's Medicaid program per State resident in FY 2010, an amount nearly 20 percent greater than that of Vermont, the State with the second highest per resident Federal Medicaid contribution, and more than 60 percent greater than the median per resident Federal Medicaid contribution.

TABLE 1—PER RESIDENT MEDICAID SPENDING (FY 2010), BY SERVICE

Geographic area	Acute care	Long-term care	DSH	Total
New York	$1,404	$1,122	$161	$2,687
California	$728	$343	$58	$1,129
	(1.93)	(3.28)	(2.78)	(2.38)
Pennsylvania	$873	$536	$66	$1,476
	(1.61)	(2.09)	(2.42)	(1.82)
USA	$805	$396	$57	$1,258
	(1.74)	(2.83)	(2.82)	(2.14)

The Committee chose the states of California and Pennsylvania to compare to New York because California is the largest state and has the second largest Medicaid program, and Pennsylvania borders New York and also has a large population USA represents national figures for the U S states plus the District of Columbia

Source Data is from the Kaiser Family Foundation

Table 2 shows how much certain states spend on Medicaid divided by the number of individuals in the state who have income below the poverty line. The numbers in parentheses show how many dollars New York spends on Medicaid for every dollar spent by the three other regions, divided by the number of people in poverty. Although a significant amount of Medicaid spending is for individuals above the poverty line, Table 2 provides perspective about State Medicaid spending relative to the number of individuals at or below the poverty line. Table 2 shows that New York's Medicaid expenditures exceed $18,000 for each person in poverty, well over double the corresponding figure for both California and the entire country, and 62 percent more than the corresponding figure for Pennsylvania. The disparity is especially pronounced for spending on long-term care services, on which New York spends more than three times what California spends and nearly three times what the country spends.

---

[9] DSH spending is intended to benefit hospitals that treat a large number of uninsured patients and patients with Medicaid. *See* Congressional Research Service, Medicaid Disproportionate Share Hospital Payments, December 18, 2012, available at http://www.fas.org/sgp/crs/misc/R42865.pdf.

TABLE 2—MEDICAID SPENDING PER PERSON IN POVERTY (FY 2010), BY SERVICE

Geographic area	Acute care	Long-term care	DSH	Total
New York	$9,653	$7,716	$1,105	$18,473
California	$4,701	$2,213	$373	$7,287
	(2.05)	(3.49)	(2.96)	(2.54)
Pennsylvania	$6,737	$4,137	$512	$11,386
	(1.43)	(1.87)	(2.16)	(1.62)
Rest of USA	$5,385	$2,654	$380	$8,419
	(1.79)	(2.91)	(2.91)	(2.19)

USA represents national figures for the U S states plus the District of Columbia
Source Data is from the Kaiser Family Foundation

Table 3 offers another comparison that demonstrates how New York spends significantly more through Medicaid, and particularly on elderly and disabled enrollees, compared to other States.

TABLE 3—MEDICAID SPENDING PER ENROLLEE (FY 2009)

Geographic area	Aged	Disabled	Adults	Children	Overall
New York	$22,494	$29,881	$4,277	$2,505	$8,960
California	10,528	16,269	1,073	1,567	3,527
	(2.14)	(1.84)	(3.99)	(1.60)	(2.54)
Pennsylvania	21,268	12,883	3,692	2,748	7,397
	(1.06)	(2.32)	(1.16)	(0.91)	(1.21)
USA	13,149	2,900	15,840	2,305	5,527
	(1.71)	(1.89)	(1.47)	(1.09)	(1.62)

USA represents national figures for the U S states plus the District of Columbia
Source Data is from the Kaiser Family Foundation

III. EXAMPLES OF PROBLEMS IN NEW YORK'S MEDICAID PROGRAM

State and Federal entities and media organizations have all found problems in the past regarding wasteful spending in New York's Medicaid program. In 2003, then-president of the United Hospital Fund, a health care policy and research organization, commented that "Medicaid became a verb—to Medicaid." [10] According to the New York Times, up to and including Governor Pataki, New York governors treated Medicaid like a political tool to get additional money from Washington.[11] Last year, the New York Times quoted Paul Castellani, former Director with New York's Office of Mental Retardation and Developmental Disabilities and now a public service professor at Rockefeller College in Albany,[12] that since 1966, New York took an aggressive approach, typified by the budget division's mantra: "[i]f it moves, Medicaid it; if it doesn't, depreciate it." [13] This historical State-approach to Medicaid financing may be a reason for the State misspending tens of billions of Federal tax dollars over the past few decades.

During the administration of Governor George E. Pataki, James Mehmet, a former chief Medicaid investigator in New York City, estimated that at least ten percent of New York City's Medicaid

---

[10] Joyce Purnick, 'Medicaid' as a Verb, Then a Crutch, New York Times (July 18, 2005), available at: http://www.nytimes.com/2003/02/24/nyregion/metro-matters-medicaid-as-a-verb-then-a-crutch.html
[11] Id.
[12] Paul J. Castellani, is also the author of From Snake Pits to Cash Cows, which was published in 2005 and details the continued operation of developmental centers in the State and its implications on Medicaid policymaking.
[13] Nina Bernstein, Cuomo's Medicaid Changes Are at Washington's Mercy, New York Times (October 23, 2012), available at: http://www.nytimes.com/2012/10/24/nyregion/new-yorks-medicaid-program-is-at-the-mercy-of-washington.html?pagewanted=all&_r=0.

spending was lost on fraudulent claims, while another 20 percent to 30 percent was misspent on unnecessary services.[14] In 2005, the New York Times criticized New York's Medicaid program for "misspending billions of dollars annually because of fraud, waste, and profiteering" after a year-long investigation into the State's program.[15] According to the Times, State oversight authorities failed to detect egregious examples of fraud in the Medicaid program, such as a dentist who billed Medicaid for 991 procedures in a single day and a Buffalo school district that rubber-stamped 4,434 special education students—nearly 60 percent of the district's special education population—onto the Medicaid rolls in a single day.[16]

These problems were mainly undetected or unacted upon by the State prior to the Times article. Moreover, the Times investigation revealed that New York had virtually no oversight of its Medicaid program at the time.[17] In 2005, largely in reaction to the Times investigation, Governor Pataki issued an executive order creating the Office of the Medicaid Inspector General (OMIG), and he appointed New York's first Medicaid inspector general.[18] In 2006, the New York State legislature codified the executive order. In April 2007, in a statement nominating James Sheehan to be Medicaid Inspector General, Governor Eliot Spitzer said, "New York State's health care spending is the highest in the nation and our system requires dramatic reform." [19]

Over the past decade, the Office of the Inspector General (OIG) for the U.S. Department of Health and Human Services (HHS) found ten specific instances in which New York State received improper Federal Medicaid payments in excess of $50 million, with six of these instances exceeding $170 million.[20] Each of these OIG reports pointed out problems in New York's Medicaid program, but New York State, under both Republican and Democratic governors, disagreed with the OIG's findings in all ten reports.[21] In 2009, New York reached a settlement with the Federal Government over false reimbursement claims for speech therapy services delivered in New York schools, which was the subject of one of the OIG reports.[22] New York agreed to pay the Federal Government $540 million to settle the lawsuit, which was filed under the Federal False Claims Act.[23] Although the $540 million amount is the largest Medicaid recovery in history, the State believed that the settlement was ap-

[14] Clifford J. Levy and Michael Luo, New York Medicaid Fraud May Reach Into Billions, New York Times (July 18, 2005), available at: http://www.nytimes.com/2005/07/18/nyregion/18medicaid.html?pagewanted=all&_r=0.

[15] Id.

[16] Id.

[17] Id.

[18] Brian McGuire, Pataki Appoints Inspector General to Oversee Medicaid Program Reform, New York Sun (July 20, 2005) available at: http://www.nysun.com/new-york/pataki-appoints-inspector-general-to-oversee/17291/.

[19] Paul Davies, Gov. Spitzer Snags Top Health-Care Fraud Buster, Law Blog, Wall Street Journal (April 6, 2007), available at: http://blogs.wsj.com/law/2007/04/06/gov-spitzer-snags-top-health-care-fraud-buster/.

[20] Schedule of Federal Produced Audits and Monetary Recommendations 01/01/2001–04/30/2012, Office of the Inspector General at the Department of Health and Human Services.

[21] Id.

[22] Nicholas Confessore, City and State Agree to Repay U.S. for Improper Medicaid Claims, New York Times (July 21, 2009), available at: http://www.nytimes.com/2009/07/22/nyregion/22whistle.html.

[23] Id.

proximately $1 billion less than what the State would have poten-
tially had to pay if the matter had gone to litigation.[24]

The following examples highlight a sampling of waste, fraud,
abuse, and mismanagement in New York State's Medicaid program
that have been highlighted or uncovered by the Committee:

*1. Lack of controls and misspending in New York City's Personal
Care Services Medicaid program* [25]

In 2009, Dr. Gabriel Feldman, a local medical director employed
by the New York County Health Services Review Organization,
filed a Federal lawsuit against the City of New York under the
False Claims Act alleging fraud, abuse, and misspending within
the Personal Care Services (PCS) program.[26] The PCS program,
which cost up to $150,000 per enrollee per year, was designed to
provide qualifying Medicaid beneficiaries services such as cleaning,
shopping, grooming and basic aid.[27] The United States Attorney for
the Southern District of New York joined Dr. Feldman's lawsuit, alleging that "the City improperly authorized and reauthorized 24-
hour care for a substantial percentage of the thousands of Medicaid
beneficiaries enrolled in the PCS program" by disregarding the requirements for enrollment.[28] According to Timothy Wyant, the expert hired by the U.S. Attorney's Office to calculate the measure
of fraud, the total damages caused by the City's conduct ranged
from $990 million to $2.581 billion using conservative assump-
tions.[29] The City of New York eventually settled this lawsuit with
the Federal Government for $70 million.[30]

2. Overpayments to New York developmental centers

In May 2012, the OIG released a report [31] that found developmental centers in the State received nearly $1.7 billion in Medicaid
payments beyond the facilities' reported costs in state fiscal year
(SFY) 2009 alone.[32] In September 2012, the Committee released a
majority staff report motivated by the OIG report showing an estimate that New York State received roughly $15 billion in excess
of reasonable costs over the past two decades from large Federal
Medicaid over-payments received by certain State-operated institutions that treat and house patients with developmental disabilities.[33] (This estimate calculates the difference between what Medicaid paid and the Committee's estimate of what Medicare would

---

[24] Id.
[25] For more information about Personal Care Services in New York and Dr. Feldman's testimony before the Committee, *See* Committee Staff Report *supra* note 1.
[26] First Amended Complaint-In-Intervention of Plaintiff-Intervenor United States of America,
United States of America ex. rel. Dr. Gabriel Feldman v. The City of New York, 09 Civ. 8381
(JSR) (S.D.N.Y. 2011).
[27] Daniel R. Levinson, HHS OIG Review of Personal Services Claims Made by Providers in
New York (A–02–07–01054), Office of the Inspector General, U.S. Department of Health and
Human Services (June 3, 2009), available at: http://www.oig.hhs gov/oas/reports/region2/
20701054.pdf.
[28] Id.
[29] First Amended Complaint-in-Intervention, Expert Report of Timothy Wyant, Ph D, *supra*
note 26 at 4.
[30] Anemona Hartocollis, City to Pay $70 Million in Medicaid Suit, N.Y. Times, Oct. 31, 2011.
[31] Medicaid Rates for NY State-Operated Developmental Centers May Be Excessive (A–02–11–
01029), Office of the Inspector General, U.S. Department of Health and Human Services (2012),
available at: http://oig.hhs.gov/oas/reports/region2/21101029.pdf [hereinafter OIG Report].
[32] According to the OIG Report, New York claimed Medicaid reimbursement totaling
$2,266,625,233 in SFY 2009 and the State's actual costs for the developmental centers that year
totaled $577,684,725. *See* id.
[33] Staff Report, The Federal Government's Failure to Prevent and End Medicaid Overpayments, U.S. House Committee on Oversight & Gov't Reform (September 20, 2012).

have paid for these patients, which is the legal allowable limit. The calculation is explained in Appendix C). The minority, while not independently verifying the methodology, agrees the figure is in the billions of dollars.

Although these facilities housed roughly 1,700 patients in 2009, total Medicaid payments to New York's developmental centers were nearly equal to the total payments Indiana's Medicaid program made for long-term care services during that year and were greater than the total Medicaid long-term care expenditures of 36 states.[34] In SFY 2011, these State-operated developmental centers in New York charged the Medicaid program $5,118 per patient per day, or the equivalent of $1.9 million per year, for a single patient.[35] One former New York State official dubbed developmental center residents "cash cows" because of the excessive payments received by the State on behalf of the residents.[36]

In 1991, Elin Howe, the then-Commissioner of the New York State Office of Mental Retardation and Developmental Disabilities, and New York Governor Mario Cuomo called for the closure of New York State developmental centers by 2000.[37] According to Howe, "[i]ndependent fiscal analyses of closure demonstrate that it is the most cost-effective course to take." [38] Former New York State Senator Nicholas A. Spano, then-Chairman of the Committee on Mental Hygiene, concurred, recommending that "all developmental centers in the State of New York be permanently closed by the year 2000." [39] However, Governor Pataki scrapped the plan to close the developmental centers by 2000, in large part because the centers generated so much revenue for the State.[40]

The payment rates ratcheted up so high because of a formula New York first negotiated with the Centers for Medicare and Medicaid Services (CMS), formerly the Health Care Financing Administration, in 1984 and then amended several times since.[41] The payment rate formula includes a factor that allows the developmental centers to maintain nearly two-thirds of the payment for a patient after the patient leaves the facility.[42] Since most of the individuals moving out of the developmental centers transition into another setting financed by Medicaid, taxpayers are effectively paying twice for individuals who leave the developmental centers.[43] In addition, CMS believes that the developmental center payments exceeded Medicaid upper payment limits established by Congress.[44]

---

[34] Kaiser Family Foundation, Distribution of Medicaid Spending by Service, FY 2010, available at: http://www.statehealthfacts.org/comparetable jsp?typ=4&ind=178&cat=4&sub=47.

[35] See OIG Report, supra note 31.

[36] Mary Beth Pfeiffer, State won't release Wassaic resident data, Poughkeepsie Journal (Oct. 29, 2010), available at: http://www.poughkeepsiejournal.com/article/20101029/NEWS01/106070006/State-won-t-release-Wassaic-resident-data.

[37] Mary Beth Pfeiffer, At $4,556 A Day, N.Y. Disabled Care No. 1 in Nation, Poughkeepsie Journal (June 20, 2010), available at: http://www.poughkeepsiejournal.com/article/20100620/NEWS01/6200374/At-4-556-day-N-Y-disabled-care-No-1-nation.

[38] Id.

[39] Id.

[40] See supra note 13.

[41] Examining the Administration's Failure to Prevent and End Medicaid Overpayments: Hearing Before the H. Comm. on Oversight & Gov't Reform, 112th Cong. (2012) (testimony of Penny Thompson, Deputy Director, Center for Medicaid and CHIP Services).

[42] See OIG Report supra note 31.

[43] See supra note 33.

[44] "[T]he Upper Payment Limit is the maximum a given State Medicaid program may pay a type of provider in the aggregate, Statewide in Medicaid fee-for-service. State Medicaid programs cannot claim Federal matching dollars for provider payments in excess of the applicable

Continued

CMS shares a large share of the blame for permitting the overpayments to rise. According to OIG:

> CMS did not adequately consider the impact of State plan amendments on the developmental centers' Medicaid daily rate. Specifically, CMS approved more than 35 State Plan Amendments related to the . . . rates, including some that pertained only to developmental centers. CMS reviewed the proposed amendments and, in some cases, asked the State for additional information to address concerns CMS had about the rate-setting methodology. However, CMS's efforts did not prevent the rate from increasing to its current level.[45]

At a 2012 Committee hearing on these overpayments, CMS agreed that the payment rates were "excessive and unacceptable" and committed to reducing the payment rates to "about one-fifth of its current level."[46] While CMS's admission was a positive sign, it only occurred after the media and the Committee shed light on decades of Federal overpayments in excess of reasonable costs and argued strongly that these rates should be immediately corrected.[47]

3. Abuses of Medicaid eligibility rules in New York

While Medicaid is commonly considered a program for the poor, middle-class and upper-class individuals often qualify for Medicaid long-term care benefits.[48] Although not specific to New York, David Armor and Sonia Sousa of George Mason University have found that nearly 80 percent of the non-disabled elderly population on Medicaid is above the poverty line, and about half of this population is over 200 percent of the poverty line.[49]

A legal industry, dubbed "Medicaid estate planning," helps Medicaid applicants and their children shelter savings and future inheritances by creatively arranging applicants' finances to meet Medicaid eligibility rules. Medicaid estate planning, a nationwide phenomenon, has been prevalent in New York State for some time, as Ned Regan, the former State Comptroller in New York, explained in a 1996 article in City Journal:

> At an unknown cost, middle- and even upper-income families often take advantage of these Medicaid services to avoid the major costs of caring for their elders. To qualify for Medicaid, middle-income people often feign poverty by placing money in a trust, by transferring assets to children or a spouse, and by preserving in their own name only assets not counted in eligibility tests—houses and cars.

UPL. . . . To create an upper bound to Medicaid spending on fee-for-service hospital rates, Congress imposed an Upper Payment Limit based on what Medicare would have paid facilities for the same services." (See Kip Piper, Medicaid Upper Payment Limits: Understanding Federal Limits on Medicaid Fee-for-Service Reimbursement of Hospitals and Nursing Homes, The Piper Report (April 25, 2012), available at: http://www.piperreport.com/blog/2012/04/25/medicaid-upper-payment-limits-understanding-federal-limits-medicaid-fee-for-service-reimbursement-hospitals-nursing-homes/.)

[45] See OIG Report, supra note 31.
[46] See supra note 41.
[47] See Committee Staff Report, supra note 1.
[48] See e g., Stephen A. Moses, Medi-Cal Long-Term Care: Safety Net or Hammock?, Pacific Research Institute (January 2011) available at: http://www.centerltc.com/pubs/Medi-Cal-LTC-SafetyNet_or_Hammock.pdf.
[49] David J. Armor and Sonia Sousa, Restoring a True Safety Net, National Affairs (Fall 2012), available at: http://www.nationalaffairs.com/publications/detail/restoring-a-true-safety-net.

These middle-class Medicaid recipients are yet another addition to Medicaid's powerful political base.[50]

Congress has attempted to reduce the problem of improper Medicaid estate planning several times over the past few decades.[51] Most recently, as part of the Deficit Reduction Act (DRA) in 2005, Congress addressed areas related to transfers of assets for less than fair market value.[52] One of the key provisions of the DRA imposed a longer look-back period, which is a period of time that states are supposed to use to review whether an individual transferred assets to another person or party for less than fair market value in order to obtain Medicaid eligibility. The DRA lengthened the look-back period from 36 months to 60 months.[53]

During a hearing on September 21, 2011, the Committee's Subcommittee on Health Care, District of Columbia, Census, and National Archives examined abuses of Medicaid eligibility rules.[54] Although the DRA has been in place for many years, Janice Eulau, assistant administrator of the Medicaid Services Division at the Suffolk County Department of Social Services, testified about the ease with which relatively wealthy New York residents, can protect their assets by enrolling in Medicaid and how roughly 60 percent of Medicaid applicants in Suffolk County [55] engage in estate planning to gain program eligibility:

> As a long-time employee of the local Medicaid office, I have had the opportunity to witness the diversion of applicants' significant resources in order to obtain Medicaid coverage. It is not at all unusual to encounter individuals and couples with resources [beyond exempt resources] exceeding $500,000, some with over $1 million. There is no attempt to hide that this money exists; there is no need. There are various legal means to prevent those funds from being used to pay for the applicant's nursing home care. Wealthy applicants for Medicaid's nursing home coverage consider that benefit to be their right, regardless of their ability to pay themselves. . . . [I]ndividuals with resources above and beyond the level prescribed by law should not be allowed to fund their children's inheritance while the taxpayers fund their nursing home care. I strongly believe that this is not a partisan issue. I also believe in the merits of the Medicaid program, but feel just as deeply that

---

[50] Ned Regan, Medicaid's Fatal Attraction, City Journal (Winter 1996), available at: http://www.city-journal.org/html/6_1_medicaids_fatal.html.

[51] For example, prior to the Deficit Reduction Act, Congress passed the Omnibus Budget Reconciliation Act (OBRA) in 1993. One of the key provisions of OBRA, which had a few provisions to address the problem of Medicaid estate planning, was to require States to recover Medicaid spending on behalf of beneficiaries from their estates after death.

[52] Centers for Medicare and Medicaid Services, Important Facts for State Policymakers: Deficit Reduction Act (January 8, 2008), available at: http://www.cms.gov/Regulations-and-Guidance/Legislation/DeficitReductionAct/downloads/TOAbackgrounder.pdf.

[53] Id.

[54] Examining Abuses of Medicaid Eligibility Rules: Hearing Before the H. Comm. on Oversight & Gov't Reform, 112th Cong. (2011).

[55] Between 2007 and 2011, median household income was $87,187 in Suffolk County compared to a median household income of $56,951 in the State. Between 2007 and 2011, 5.7% of persons in Suffolk County were below the poverty level compared to 14.5% of people in the State. *See* United States Census Bureau, U.S. Dep't. of Commerce, State and County Quick Facts, Suffolk County New York, available at: http://quickfacts.census.gov/qfd/states/36/36103.html (last visited February 2013).

these issues regarding resource diversion need to be addressed.[56]

Eulau also testified about a technique called "spousal refusal," a provision of the Medicare Catastrophic Coverage Act of 1988 that is being misused in New York.[57] Under spousal refusal, a couple shifts assets from a sick or disabled spouse to a healthy spouse in order to "artificially impoverish" the sick or disabled spouse and qualify him or her for Medicaid. The healthy spouse then invokes spousal refusal and declines to provide financial support for the spouse who is on Medicaid.[58] Moreover, under spousal refusal, income earned by the healthy spouse is exempt from being considered available to the impoverished spouse.

According to the New York Times, "[w]hile many state and local governments do not openly acknowledge the spousal refusal option, New York City actually provides a form letter for it." [59] In 2009, more than 1,200 people in New York City invoked spousal refusal, a significant increase from prior years.[60] The Times article also indicated that the City reviewed spousal refusal applications to recover money, but only $3.7 million was recovered in 2009, or less than $3,000 on average for each individual invoking spousal refusal.[61] Eulau testified that most married people in Suffolk County, New York, who apply for Medicaid use spousal refusal, and she confirmed to Committee staff that the use of this technique has grown over time.[62] Governor Cuomo's recently introduced 2013–2014 executive budget proposes the elimination of spousal refusal with an estimated annual State savings of $137 million.[63]

4. Excessive salaries paid to executives of Medicaid-funded organizations

The Committee has found that Federal taxpayers have subsidized lavish lifestyles for many executives in organizations that receive almost all of their funding through Medicaid. The Committee's oversight work in this area was informed by an August 2011 New York Times article that exposed how top executives at the Young Adult Institute (YAI)—a nonprofit that runs group homes for the developmentally disabled—used Medicaid funds to lease luxury cars, to pay tuition bills and living expenses for their children, and to reward themselves with generous compensation packages.[64] In fact, four executives at the YAI (Phillip Levy, Joel Levy, Tom Dern, and Stephen Freeman) each received compensation in

---

[56] Examining Abuses of Medicaid Eligibility Rules: Hearing Before the H. Comm. on Oversight & Gov't Reform, 112th Cong. (2011) (testimony of Janice Eulau, Assistant Administrator for Medicaid, Suffolk County, New York Department of Social Services).

[57] Id.

[58] Allan Rubin and Harold Rubin, Spousal Refusal to Pay for Nursing Home Costs, therubins.com (Feb. 7, 2009), available at: http://www.therubins.com/legal/refusal.htm.

[59] Anemona Hartocollis, Full Wallets, but Using Health Program for Poor, New York Times (December 10, 2010), available at: http://www.nytimes.com/2010/12/12/nyregion/12medicaid.html?pagewanted=all.

[60] Id.

[61] Id.

[62] See supra note 56.

[63] New York State 2013–2014 Executive Budget Matrix, (viewed February 12, 2013), available at: http://www.health.ny.gov/health_care/medicaid/redesign/docs/2013-14_exec_budget_matrix.xls

[64] Russ Beuttner, Reaping Millions in Nonprofit Care for Disabled, New York Times (August 2, 2011), available at: http://www.nytimes.com/2011/08/02/nyregion/for-executives-at-group-homes-generous-pay-and-little-oversight.html?pagewanted=all.

excess of $1 million in 2008, with money derived almost entirely from Medicaid.[65]

While YAI may be the worst offender, a number of Medicaid-financed organizations in New York paid exceptionally high executive salaries funded with tax revenue. A review conducted by the Committee of a sample of Medicaid-financed organizations found that at least 15 executives received yearly compensation exceeding $500,000 and more than 100 other executives received yearly compensation exceeding $200,000 per year.[66] The Committee's study was not a comprehensive or exhaustive search of compensation packages received by top employees at Medicaid-funded organizations, but rather a simple search of publicly available IRS 990 Forms for 2008 and 2011.

IV. PATIENT ABUSE WITHIN THE DEVELOPMENTALLY DISABLED SYSTEM IN NEW YORK

In 2011 and 2012, the New York Times ran a series titled— 'Abused and Used' chronicling how the large expenditures New York's Medicaid program do not necessarily translate into quality care received by the developmentally disabled.[67] For example, despite the large payments received by the State for the residents of developmental centers, the Times reported that patient care is often substandard:

> [T]he institutions are hardly a model: Those who run them have tolerated physical and psychological abuse, knowingly hired unqualified workers, ignored complaints by whistle-blowers and failed to credibly investigate cases of abuse and neglect, according to a review by The New York Times of thousands of state records and court documents, along with interviews of current and former employees. Since 2005, seven of the institutions have failed inspections by the State Health Department, which oversees the safety and living conditions of the residents.[68]

According to the New York Times, New York State consistently failed to take complaints from employees of the developmental centers or family members of residents seriously.[69] According to the Times, employees who reported problems experienced retaliation by other employees, and the length of time it took to settle complaints disincentivized employees from filing complaints in the first place.[70] According to the Times, a number of residents suffered significant verbal, emotional, and physical abuse at the developmental centers.[71] Several residents at New York's developmental centers, and at numerous Medicaid-financed group homes across the State, have died directly because of employee incompetence or negligence,

---

[65] This information obtained from publicly available 990 forms.

[66] See Appendix B for Committee's data on salaries for executives at nonprofits funded by Medicaid in New York State.

[67] See Abused and Used, New York Times, available at http://www.nytimes.com/interactive/nyregion/abused-and-used-series-page.html.

[68] Danny Hakim, A Disabled Boy's Death, and a System in Disarray, New York Times (June 5, 2011), available at: http://www.nytimes.com/2011/06/06/nyregion/boys-death-highlights-crisis-in-homes-for-disabled.html?pagewanted=all&_r=0.

[69] Id.

[70] Id.

[71] See supra note 67.

and in some cases even from manslaughter at the hands of their caretakers.[72]

The Poughkeepsie Journal reported that a large part of the problem of poor resident care appears to be the difficulty of firing incompetent or neglectful employees:

> Since 2007, the state has tried to fire employees of a dozen local facilities for the developmentally disabled 20 times. It has failed 18 times. Quite simply, it's nearly impossible to get fired from state-run facilities that care for people with autism, Down Syndrome and other mental disabilities, according to a Poughkeepsie Journal review of 1,900 pages of disciplinary documents involving 98 group homes and six institutions statewide. Just 2 percent of cases resulted in termination, with workers keeping jobs even in cases of serious alleged abuse and neglect.[73]

The Poughkeepsie Journal found that workers who left disabled people alone in a running vehicle or outside in the rain kept their jobs. Additionally, workers who stole State property, brought drug paraphernalia to work, or harassed disabled residents almost always kept their jobs.[74] An article in the New York Times suggests that the Civil Service Employees Association (CSEA) is partially to blame for this problem.[75] According to the New York Times, "the union's approach—contesting just about every charge leveled at a worker—contributed to a system in which firings of even the most abusive employees are rare." [76] Office of People with Developmental Disabilities (OPWDD) former spokesman Herm Hill said OPWDD's hands were often tied in cases against abusive workers because of the disciplinary and arbitration rules involving the workers' union.[77] The union's representation of repeat offenders made it possible for employees to rack up serious offenses before losing their jobs.[78]

V. PAST HEALTH-CARE-RELATED CORRUPTION BY ELECTED OFFICIALS

In the last decade, at least half a dozen elected State representatives, including two State Senate Majority leaders, have been convicted of theft, bribery, or honest services fraud,[79] related to health care:

• On May 14, 2012, former New York State Senate Majority Leader Pedro Espada was convicted in Federal court on four counts of theft for stealing over $500,000 from Soundview, the nonprofit health care network he founded in the Bronx which received Federal funding in excess of $1 million per year.[80] Federal Medicaid

---

[72] Id.

[73] Mary Beth Pfeiffer, Caregivers of Mentally Disabled Keep Jobs, even in cases of abuse, neglect, Poughkeepsie Journal (September 17, 2011), available at: http://www.poughkeepsiejournal.com/article/20110918/PROMO/109180384/Journal-investigation-Caregivers-mentally-disabled-keep-jobs-even-cases-abuse-neglect.

[74] Id.

[75] Danny Hakim, At State-Run Homes, Abuse and Impunity, New York Times (March 12, 2011), available at: http://www.nytimes.com/2011/03/13/nyregion/13homes.html?pagewanted=all.

[76] Id.

[77] Id.

[78] Id.

[79] Honest services fraud is Federal crime defined in Skilling v. United States as "fraudulent schemes to deprive another of honest services through bribes or kickbacks supplied by a third party who has not been deceived." (Skilling v. United States 130 S. Ct. 2896, (2010))

[80] Espada is expected to face a retrial on four other counts of theft, fraud and conspiracy on which the jury failed to agree after his six-week trial. See Mosi Secret, Ex-State Senator Guilty

money that was intended to be used for health care for the city's poorest residents instead paid for private family parties, school tuition, luxury car payments and $100,000 in lobster, sushi and other meals.[81] Additionally, Espada packed the Soundview board and staff with members of his own family and close personal friends.[82]

• In May of 2012, former New York Senate Majority Leader Joseph Bruno was charged with two counts of fraud for accepting $440,000 from a businessman who managed the assets of a health and welfare fund and sought the then-Senator's influence in legislative matters.[83]

• Former New York State Senator Carl Kruger was sentenced to seven years in prison after pleading guilty to two counts of conspiracy to commit honest services fraud [84] and two counts of conspiracy to commit bribery.[85] Mr. Kruger accepted bribes from two hospital executives, a prominent lobbyist and a healthcare consultant in exchange for taking official action on behalf of those parties, including sponsoring and supporting legislation, favorably directing state grants, and writing to State officials in his capacity as State legislator.[86]

• In 2005, former New York State Senator Guy Velella pled guilty to one count of bribery and was sentenced to one year in prison for the felony conviction.[87] He was charged with a 25-count indictment alleging the solicitation of $250,000 in bribes for steering public works contracts to those who paid the bribes.[88] During the 1990s, his law firm was given hundreds of thousands of dollars in legal work by large insurance companies while he headed the State Senate Committee that oversaw legislation affecting them.[89]

• In 2004, New York State Assemblyman Anthony Seminerio pled guilty to a single fraud count for influence peddling and was sentenced to six years in prison.[90] Seminerio admitted to promoting the interests of Jamaica Hospital Medical Center, from which he received over $300,000 for obtaining State financing and lobbying

of Theft from Nonprofit, New York Times (May 14, 2012), available at: http://www.nytimes.com/2012/05/15/nyregion/ex-senator-espada-guilty-of-embezzling-from-soundview-health-network.html?pagewanted=all.

[81] Id.

[82] Julia Marsh and Dan Mangan, Pedro's board stiffs were his puppets, New York Post (March 21, 2012), available at: http://www.nypost.com/p/news/local/bronx/pedro_board_stiffs_EjyOnu7lWNZZyXtXqtzpBM.

[83] Joseph L. Bruno, Times Topics, New York Times (updated May 4, 2012) available at http://topics.nytimes.com/top/reference/timestopics/people/b/joseph_l_bruno/index.html?inline=nyt-per ("The indictment, unsealed in Federal District Court in Albany, came nearly six months after a Federal appeals court vacated Mr. Bruno's previous conviction because of a ruling in a separate case by the United States Supreme Court that undermined the government's legal claims against Mr. Bruno, a Republican from Rensselaer County. But the appeals court said Mr. Bruno could be retried on different charges.")

[84] See supra note 79.

[85] Benjamin Weiser, Former State Senator Is Sentenced to 7 Years in Vast Bribery Case, New York Times (April 26, 2012), available at: http://www.nytimes.com/2012/04/27/nyregion/carl-kruger-sentenced-to-seven-years-in-corruption-case.html.

[86] Id.

[87] Liz Krueger, Former Senator Guy Velella: Convicted Felon, $80,000-A-Year Public Pensioner, Gotham Gazette (October 25, 2004), available at: http://www.gothamgazette.com/article/fea/20041025/202/1156.

[88] Id.

[89] Clifford J. Levy and Christopher Drew, In Albany, Ally of Insurers Profits From Them, New York Times (February 4, 2011), available at: http://www.nytimes.com/2001/02/04/nyregion/in-albany-ally-of-insurers-profits-from-them.html.

[90] David M. Halbfinger and William Rashbaum, Ex-Assemblyman From Queens Dies In Federal Prison, New York Times (January 7, 2011), available at: http://query.nytimes.com/gst/fullpage.html?res=9D02EFD7143AF934A35752C0A9679D8B63.

legislators on behalf of the hospital's efforts to take over other hospitals.[91]

Outright corruption and favoritism has occurred in New York. For example, Kenneth Bruno, son of former New York State Senate Majority Leader Joseph Bruno, was hired as a lobbyist for the New York Ambulette Coalition on the same day that the State Legislature eliminated $4.4 million in Medicaid transportation funding that would have gone to the Coalition's members.[92] Within ten days, the funding was restored "at the insistence of the Senate," according to a senior State official.[93] Bruno reportedly called his father's top aides personally to ask them to restore the funds.[94] Leaders throughout New York State voiced their disapproval about Bruno's lobbying deal. Conservative Party Leader Michael Long said the deal "shows the system is broken," and Rachel Leon, executive director of Common Cause, called the action by Bruno's son "an instant symbol of what's wrong in Albany." [95]

VI. ALLEGATIONS OF PROBLEMS WITH STATE OVERSIGHT OF THE MEDICAID PROGRAM

Several whistle-blowers within the New York State health care system have brought to light serious failures indicating that the State bureaucracy historically failed to adequately police Medicaid waste, fraud and abuse. Paul F. Stavis, counsel to three different New York State health agencies during his 28-year career, alleged that "anti-fraud efforts in New York have not been taken seriously by the State's executive agencies." [96] In an April 2011 article in Newsday, Stavis cited multiple examples of Medicaid-related fiscal abuse [97] and how both the State's Department of Health (DOH) and the State's Office of the Medicaid Inspector General (OMIG) looked the other way when faced with evidence of Medicaid fraud.[98]

According to Stavis, New York State continued to pay providers who were suspected of abusing the Medicaid system. For instance, the DOH gave a $1 million grant to Pedro Espada's nonprofit, Soundview, even after seeing evidence of ongoing fraud.[99] In fact, Stavis brought evidence of Espada's illegal activities to the attention of the DOH in 2005 and OMIG in 2007, years before the

---

[91] Id.

[92] Fredric U. Dicker, It Pays (4.4 million) to Hire Bruno's Son, New York Post (April 25, 2005), available at: http://www.nypost.com/p/news/item_Usy1VfKTPyNavkRCN2mb4K.

[93] Id.

[94] Id.

[95] Fredric U. Dicker, Pol Son Burned—Right & Left Agree: Bruno Kin's Deal Is Wrong, New York Post (April 26, 2005), available at: http://www.nypost.com/p/news/item_IwRwuubUpAd1M23lYXtDCK.

[96] Paul Stavis, NY too weak on Medicaid fraud, Newsday (April 1, 2011), available at: http://www.newsday.com/opinion/oped/stavis-ny-too-weak-on-medicaid-fraud-1.2795786.

[97] See id. Stavis states that New York State law contains a loophole that prevents the State from prosecuting certain types of Medicaid fraud, which then necessitates the Federal Government's intervention when such misappropriation crimes are committed. Stavis characterized the inability of New York State to prosecute and the resulting need for Federal involvement as an "embarrassment." Although Stavis drafted legislation to close the loophole during his tenure as counsel for the State, Stavis writes that the New York State legislature refused to pass this legislation.

[98] Id. In addition to outright fraudulent activities, New York State historically has had numerous cases of fiscal abuse regarding Medicaid. In an outstanding example of fiscal abuse, Stavis cites instances where providers diverted Medicaid funds to make donations to charities in foreign countries, give nearly $2 million per year to a house of worship, fund religious schools, and pay excessively high salaries to executives at nonprofit corporations.

[99] Jacob Gershman, State Ignored Call to Probe Espada Clinics, Wall Street Journal (December 17, 2010), available at: http://online.wsj.com/article/SB100014240527 4870339520457602384335249746.html.

former State Senate Majority leader was convicted of Medicaid fraud. No action was taken by either State office.[100] The illegal payments continued until 2011, when the Federal Government ordered the payments stopped and commenced criminal proceedings against Espada.[101]

Earlier, this report highlighted the suit Dr. Gabriel Feldman brought against the City of New York in 2009.[102] As a medical director, Feldman determined which individuals met the qualifications for Medicaid-funded home health care services. Despite firm criteria outlining program eligibility, Feldman encountered "tremendous pressure" from advocacy groups, politicians, and family members of clients to approve service requests for individuals who did not meet the qualifications.[103] When he refused to grant such requests, Feldman found that his decisions were "knowingly, intentionally and routinely being overridden without legal basis" [104] in order "to admit as many clients as possible who apply for the PCS Program regardless of his or her condition, fitness or qualification for the program." [105] In testimony before the Committee, Feldman stated that pre-2011 "a pervasive culture of non-accountability and non-compliance to PCS State regulations made it simply far too easy for local social service offices in New York City to spend billions in taxpayer money without regard to common sense oversight, regulations of the State, or patient safety concerns." [106]

During the Committee's hearing, Feldman used the term "Medicaid industrial complex" [107] to refer "to the New York State Government, the healthcare providers and the unions essentially operating as one unified entity and making any enforcement and recovery actions largely unsuccessful." [108] Feldman further explained that the pre-2011 "system of quality assurance, oversight, and rate setting was completely dysfunctional" and there were and still are "insufficient resources and staff in the [Medicaid] Inspector General's Office and in New York City's Human Resource Administration, devoted to enforcing fiscal discipline and fraud oversight in the system." [109] Like Stavis, Feldman also indicts the DOH for having "utterly failed in their oversight functions." [110]

VII. REFORMS IN THE LAST TWO YEARS AND ADDITIONAL CONCERNS

During his first month as New York's Governor, Andrew Cuomo called for Medicaid reform, stating, "New York's bloated Medicaid program, which spends at a rate more than twice the national average, must be reformed to help our state begin to make ends

---

[100] Id.
[101] See Stavis, *supra* note 96.
[102] Is Government Adequately Protecting Taxpayers from Medicaid Fraud?: Hearing Before the H. Comm. on Oversight & Gov't Reform, 112th Cong. (2012) (testimony of Gabriel Feldman, Local Medical Director, New York Personal Care Services Program).
[103] Id.
[104] First Amended Complaint-In-Intervention of Plaintiff-Intervenor United States of America, United States of America ex. rel. Dr. Gabriel Feldman v. The City of New York, 09 Civ. 8381 (JSR) (S.D.N.Y. 2011).
[105] Id.
[106] See *supra* note 102.
[107] Id.
[108] Letter from Gabriel Feldman to H. Comm. on Oversight & Gov't Reform, Response to Questions for the Record (May 10, 2012) (on file with Committee).
[109] Id.
[110] Id.

meet." [111] The administration of Governor Cuomo has taken positive steps to reform some of the problems discussed in Section III and Section IV of this report. These efforts have been dubbed by the New York Post as "a break with past efforts" because of the support he obtained from the Service Employees International Union and the hospital association.[112]

New York State implemented the first-in-the-nation statutory "global" spending cap. This State spending cap imposes an annual limit on the growth of State Medicaid expenditures, not to exceed the medical Consumer Price Index. The cap remains in effect, even if the number of eligible Medicaid beneficiaries rises. In FY 2012–2013, New York experienced a 4 percent increase in Medicaid spending from the previous year, one of the nation's lowest rates of increase. New York State projects that their newly-implemented Medicaid reforms will save the Federal Government $17 billion over five years.[113]

In the first year of the Cuomo administration, the State started a phase-out of fee-for-service home care, an action which may ensure greater integrity in the PCS program. This effort began in New York City, where the State converted the City's fee-for-service PCS program to the State's Medicaid Managed Long Term Care program.[114] According to Dr. Feldman, there have been some additional measures "taken by New York City and New York State to ensure proper compliance with Federal and State regulations" for the PCS program.[115]

New York and CMS have entered negotiations about reducing the developmental center payment rate through the Medicaid State Plan Amendment process.[116] According to the Wall Street Journal, "New York has agreed to give up about $800 million in payments to the developmental centers." [117] CMS is currently reviewing a State Plan Amendment submitted by New York that would reduce the payments received by New York through the State-operated developmental centers.

On January 18, 2012, Governor Cuomo issued an executive order to address the problem of outrageous executive compensation packages at taxpayer-financed organization.[118] The order recognized that "New York has an ongoing obligation to ensure that taxpayers' dollars are used properly, efficiently and effectively to improve the lives of New Yorkers and our communities," and that "in certain instances providers of services that receive State funds or State-authorized payments have used such funds to pay for excessive administrative costs and outsized compensation for their senior ex-

[111] Governor Andrew M. Cuomo, Press Release, Governor Cuomo Issues Executive Order Creating Medicaid Redesign Team (January 5, 2011) available at http://www.governor.ny.gov/press/01052011medicaid.

[112] Id.

[113] Governor Andrew M. Cuomo, Press Release, Governor Cuomo Announces that New York Submits Federal Waiver to Invest $10 Billion in Medicaid Redesign Team Savings to Transform the State's Health Care System (August 6, 2012), available at: http://www.governor.ny.gov/press/08062012-federal-waiver-health-care.

[114] New York 2013–2014 Executive Budget, NY Rising, (January 22, 2013), available at: http://publications.budget.ny.gov/eBudget1314/fy1314littlebook/BriefingBook.pdf.

[115] See supra note 108.

[116] Laura Nahmias, Budget Hole Seen After Loss of Aid, Wall Street Journal (January 24, 2013), available at: http://online.wsj.com/article/SB10001424127887324539304578262311978071202.html.

[117] Id.

[118] Governor Andrew M. Cuomo, State of New York, Executive Order 38 (Jan. 18, 2012), available at: www.governor.ny.gov/executiveorder/38.

ecutives." [119] The Governor's order directed that payments to "providers of services that receive reimbursements directly or indirectly" from State agencies "shall not be provided for compensation paid or given to any executive by such provider in an amount greater than $199,000." [120] The Governor's order also stated: "A provider's failure to comply with such regulations established by the applicable State agency shall, in the commissioner's sole discretion, form the basis for termination or non-renewal of the agency's contract with or continued support of the provider." [121]

Governor Cuomo proposed eliminating spousal refusal in New York in his first and second budget.[122] However, powerful interest groups, especially the elder law bar, lobbied strongly to prevent the change. The interest groups' opposition proved successful, and New York did not enact legislation to end the abuse of spousal refusal.[123] In his 2013–2014 budget proposal, Governor Cuomo has again proposed changes that would reduce the ability of individuals in New York to abuse the spousal refusal technique by passing inappropriate private costs onto taxpayers.[124]

Through a series of recommendations by Cuomo's Medicaid Redesign Team and implemented by the State, New York has expanded the definition of an estate for the purpose of estate recovery. The State also centralized responsibility for Medicaid estate recovery process in OMIG. Like most States, New York has not historically been aggressive recovering from estates of individuals who utilize Medicaid to pay for their long-term care services. In 2004, only 0.8 percent of Medicaid expenditures on nursing homes was recovered nationally, and only 0.5 percent of Medicaid expenditures on nursing homes was recovered by New York.[125] The hope is that these reforms will make it easier for New York to recover from the estates of individuals who have inappropriately used Medicaid to pay for long-term care services and supports.

In 2011, after what was dubbed "an unprecedented string of corruption cases" by the Huffington Post New York,[126] the State legislature passed the Public Integrity Reform Act of 2011.[127] The new law requires members of the State legislature to accurately disclose any outside income, as well as the names of clients. It also created a new Joint Commission on Public Ethics, with the power to investigation lawmakers, their staff and members of the executive

---

[119] Id.

[120] Id.

[121] Id.

[122] Carl Campanile, Andy to end 'rich' home-care ruse, New York Post (March 7, 2011), available at: http://www.nypost.com/p/news/local/andy_to_end_rich_home_care_ruse_UO5gsIz0Fcat1zrZ1XwXdP.

[123] Sanford Altman, Better With Age: NY seniors win as Legislature drops provision, Times Herald-Record (April 10, 2012), available at: http://www.recordonline.com/apps/pbcs.dll/article?AID=/20120410/BIZ/204100328.

[124] Memorandum in Support, Health and Mental Hygiene Article VII Legislation, 2013–2014 New York State Executive Budget available at http://publications.budget.ny.gov/eBudget1314/fy1314artVIIbills/HMH_ArticleVII_MS.pdf.

[125] Medicaid Estate Recovery Collections, U.S. Department of Health and Human Services (September 2005), available at: http://aspe.hhs.gov/daltcp/reports/estreccol.htm#table1.

[126] Michael Gormley, The Clean Up Albany Act of 2011 Proposed, Huff Post New York (June 3, 2011), available at: http://www.huffingtonpost.com/2011/06/04/the-clean-up-albany-act-o_n_871329.html.

[127] Jisha V. Dymond, Governor Cuomo Signs Ethics Bill, Corporate Political Activity Law Blog (August 16, 2011), available at: http://www.corporatepoliticalactivitylaw.com/index.php/2011/08/governor-cuomo-signs-ethics-bill/.

branch for legal and ethical violations.[128] According to the New York Times, there are "questions whether the reforms would be weaker than expected." [129] For instance, the Times points out that a 12–2 vote of the new Commission in favor of an investigation could still lose.[130]

New York State is taking steps to improve the protection and safety of disabled children and adults in the State's care.[131] In 2011, Governor Cuomo appointed a special advisor, Clarence Sundram,[132] to identify gaps in care that create a potentially harmful environment for disabled persons.[133] The resulting analysis became the basis for the reforms. The Cuomo reform efforts forced the resignations of top officials in the Office for People with Developmental Disabilities (OPWDD) and the Commission on Quality of Care and Advocacy for Persons with Disabilities.[134]

New initiatives include enhanced training and recruitment and higher employment standards. Strict policies regarding abuse and neglect were adopted, with immediate suspensions of employees in substantiated cases of physical and sexual abuse. New hires now face drug testing, comprehensive background checks, and employment screening through an Excluded Provider Registry.[135]

The hope is that the reorganizing of management will better integrate services with law enforcement and separate operations from investigations.[136] All OPWDD investigators receive law enforcement investigative training, and, starting in 2012, new State police cadets receive training to support OPWDD standards.[137]

Although long overdue, New York State's current policy is to pursue termination of employees found to have committed egregious abuse and neglect of patients. OPWDD pushed for and obtained CSEA's agreement to negotiate a standardized table of penalties to remove arbitrator discretion when an employee is found to have committed a serious act of abuse or neglect. New State mandates require providers report abuse and neglect cases to law enforcement and the State, and to verify backgrounds of job applicants against a database the State will maintain.

The Cuomo administration and the New York legislature also established the Justice Center for the Protection of People with Special Needs.[138] When it is in place, the Justice Center will maintain

---

[128] Id.

[129] Danny Hakim and Thomas Kaplan, As Ethics Measure Emerges, So Do Questions About Its Teeth, New York Times (June 7, 2011), available at: http://www.nytimes.com/2011/06/08/nyregion/ny-ethics-bill-may-lack-some-teeth.html.

[130] Id.

[131] Andrew Cuomo's worthy attempt to fix shameful, dangerous state programs for the disabled, New York Daily News (May 8, 2012), available at: www.nydailynews.com/opinion/andrew-cuomo-worthy-attempt-fix-shameful-dangerous-state-programs-disabled-article-1.1074021.

[132] Sundram is a national expert on institutions and programs for the mentally disabled.

[133] Memorandum for Program Bill #35, New York Governor's Program Bill 2012, available at: www.governor.ny.gov/assets/documents/GPB35-PEOPLE-WITH-SPECIAL-NEEDS-MEMO.pdf.

[134] Danny Hakim, State Faults Care for the Disabled, New York Times (Mar. 22, 2012), available at: www.nytimes.com/2012/03/22/nyregion/new-york-state-draft-report-finds-needless-risk-in-care-for-the-disabled.html?pagewanted=all&_r=0).

[135] New York State Office of the Medicaid Inspector General, Restricted, Terminated or Excluded Individuals or Entities, available at: www.omig.state.ny.us/data/content/view/72/52/).

[136] New York Office for People With Developmental Disabilities, Commissioner's Page, available at: www.opwdd.ny.gov/opwdd_about/commissioners_page/accomplishments).

[137] New York State Office for People with Developmental Disabilities, Joint Agreement Announced Between OPWDD and State Police to Reform Abuse Reporting System (Aug 18, 2011), available at: www.opwdd.ny.gov/news_and_publications/opwdd_news/joint_agreement state_ police_abuse_reporting_system.

[138] Justice Center For the Protection of People with Special Needs, available at: www.governor.ny.gov/Justice4SpecialNeeds/home.

a 24-hour hotline to route calls regarding allegations of abuse and neglect. An in-house special prosecutor and inspector general at the Justice Center will be primarily responsible for the investigation of serious allegations of a criminal nature.[139] The Center incorporates many of the responsibilities of the defunct Commission on Quality of Care and Advocacy for Persons with Disabilities.[140]

The Committee minority is greatly encouraged by the systemic overhaul of New York State's care for the developmentally disabled led by the OPWDD. The Cuomo administration engaged new leadership to address the mismanagement plaguing the system.[141] The new OPWDD appears to be focused on real improvements with the Commissioner providing reports detailing areas of progress at the six-month, one-year and eighteen-month intervals.[142]

While those and other reforms are significant steps forward, the Committee has some ongoing concerns.

CMS first inquired about the excessive payment rates in 2010, over two-and-a-half years ago.[143] CMS and New York have finally agreed to an audit, scheduled to begin this month, to uncover the magnitude of the excessive developmental center payments. Correcting overpayments of this magnitude should not be a multi-year process.

The Committee is concerned by the lack of State cooperation with the Committee's oversight in this area. On July 19, 2012, Chairman Issa and Congressman Gowdy sent a letter to Nirav Shah, the Commissioner of New York's Department of Health requesting information related to the developmental center overpayments.[144] The Committee received indication throughout the next few weeks that the State was going to provide the requested information. However, the State ultimately decided not to cooperate with the Committee's request by citing that providing the information would not be in the State's best interests.[145] To date, the State of New York has not supplied any of the requested information to the Committee.

The Committee is also concerned by recent allegations relating to the State's OMIG, the agency tasked with "preventing and detecting fraudulent, abusive, and wasteful practices within the Medicaid program and recovering improperly expended Medicaid funds." [146] In November 2012, the Albany Times Union ran a story based largely on the reporter's interviews with ten current and former

---

[139] New York Governor Andrew Cuomo Press Office, Governor Cuomo and Legislative Leaders Announce Agreement on Legislation to Protect People with Special Needs and Disabilities (June 17, 2012), available at: www.governor.ny gov/press/061712justice4specialneedsagreement.

[140] Id.

[141] New York Governor Andrew Cuomo Press Office, Governor Cuomo Announces New Leadership for State Agencies that Serve disabled New Yorkers (Mar. 7, 2011), available at: www.governor.ny.gov/press/leadership.

[142] New York Office for People with Developmental Disabilities, Commissioner's Page, available at: www.opwdd.ny.gov/opwdd_about/commissioners_page.

[143] Letter from Sue Kelly, Associate Regional Administrator, Division of Medicaid and Children's Health, CMS to Donna Frescatore, Deputy Commissioner, NY State Department of Health, (July 13, 2010) (on file with Committee).

[144] Letter from Darrell Issa, Chairman of House Committee on Oversight and Government Reform, and Trey Gowdy, Chairman of House Committee on Oversight and Government Reform Subcommittee on Health Care, District of Columbia, Census and National Archives.

[145] Email from New York Counsel to Committee on Oversight and Government Reform staff (September 4, 2012) (on file with Committee).

[146] Office of the New York State Medicaid Inspector General, Mission Statement, available at http://www.omig ny.gov/data/content/blogcategory/20/192/

OMIG employees.[147] According to these current and former employees, New York's OMIG suffers from misdirection and its investigations lack a sense of urgency.[148] Former employees allege that OMIG has recently backed off audits and investigations of organizations suspected of Medicaid fraud and abuse for politically-motivated reasons.[149] According to the Times Union article, "One veteran employee said when factoring for the recoveries made by outside contractors, particularly one cracking down on third-party claims, the sums recovered by OMIG staff are pretty dismal.' Data from the reports [shared with the reporter] back up the contention." [150]

Articles in the Times Union and the New York Times suggest that problems began at OMIG when Governor Cuomo replaced James Sheehan, who took an aggressive approach to combating problems in the State's Medicaid program and was largely credited with recouping $1.5 billion in Medicaid overpayments in a four-year period, with James Cox, a former Regional Inspector General of the HHS OIG as Medicaid Inspector in July 2011.[151] Sheehan believes that he was removed as the Inspector General of OMIG because he represented a challenge to a powerful Medicaid industry in New York that is a large employment engine.[152] According to Sheehan, "Medicaid is to New York what corn is to Iowa. It's a heavy lift." [153] It should be noted that Paul Stavis, who also worked for Sheehan in addition to his other positions, was also critical of OMIG during Jim Sheehan's tenure stating "Fraud litigation is very difficult and expensive and OMIG has not equipped itself to cope with such cases. [OMIG doesn't] look for fraud as a matter of practice." [154]

Eight months before the Times Union article, a New York Times article reported that audits released by the State show that Cox's findings of overpayments fell steeply after September 30, 2011, the deadline for the State to meet a $1.5 billion Federal target imposed when the New York OMIG was created in 2006.[155] According to the New York Times, New York was on target to avoid $1.1 billion in the previous year.[156] Cost avoidance is an estimate of public money not spent because of education and discussions with providers. However, the Times article also pointed out that most of the important audits responsible for the avoided cost were started under Sheehan.[157]

---

[147] James M. Odato, Fraud agency called adrift: Office of Medicaid Inspector General is ineffective and mismanaged, critics say, Times Union (November 19, 2012), available at http://www.timesunion.com/local/article/Fraud-agency-called-adrift-4047131.php

[148] Id.

[149] Id.

[150] Id.

[151] See Nina Bernstein, Under Pressure, New York Moves to Soften Tough Medicaid Audits, New York Times, (March 18, 2012), available at: http://www.nytimes.com/2012/03/19/nyregion/new-medicaid-inspector-general-supports-less-adversarial-audits.html?pagewanted=all and supra note 148.

[152] See Nina Bernstein, Under Pressure, New York Moves to Soften Tough Medicaid Audits, New York Times, (March 18, 2012), available at http://www.nytimes.com/2012/03/19/nyregion/new-medicaid-inspector-general-supports-less-adversarial-audits.html?pagewanted=all.

[153] Id.

[154] Jacob Gershman, Medicaid Fraud Unit Falls Short, Wall Street Journal (January 27, 2011), available at: http://online.wsj.com/article/SB20001424052748703293204576106260159071844.html 155 See supra note 153.

[155] See supra note 153.

[156] Id.

[157] Id.

Sheehan's aggressive approach was not without controversy. According to the New York Times, the health care industry lobbied for James Sheehan's removal as New York's Medicaid Inspector General [158] and also for legislation that would limit "what are perceived to be overzealous and unfair tactics employed by OMIG in audits." [159] At a New York State legislature hearing in 2010, a lawyer for the health care industry accused Sheehan's auditors of "gangster-style tactics." [160] This legislation, which cut the government's time to reclaim overpayments in half and let providers submit corrected bills rather than repay, overwhelmingly passed the New York State legislature.[161] To Governor Cuomo's credit, he vetoed the legislation stating that "the bill seeks to make changes to the law that are too far-reaching and would potentially allow fraudulent and abuse activity to go undetected and unprosecuted." [162]

The Committee minority believes that the allegations contained in the New York Times and Albany Times Union articles are inconsistent with some of the evidence. The minority is aware that the number of OMIG investigations has remained consistent and in some cases exceeded the performance of the agency under Sheehan since the Cuomo administration's appointment of Cox. According to information in reports published by OMIG, OMIG's cost savings activities, which include avoided costs as well as recovered improper payments, rose significantly—by 34 percent in 2011, and recoveries, which totaled about $700 million in 2011, also continue to grow.[163]

The Committee minority believes that while it is too soon to tell how OMIG's recovery performance will turn out for 2012, a partial year analysis of New York Medicaid Global Cap Reports suggests that OMIG is on course to surpass that mark.[164] Using these trends, the minority believes there is not evidence in the data to substantiate the claims that OMIG is suffering under Cox's leadership.

The Committee majority staff believes it is impossible to use annual figures to characterize a trend since James Sheehan was Inspector General at OMIG for more than half of 2011 and many audits begun under Sheehan's guidance would not have resulted in recoveries until later in the year or in subsequent years.

VIII. RECOMMENDATIONS

New York's State Medicaid Plan, like almost all State Medicaid Plans, consists of thousands of pages of dense rules and reimbursement methodologies. According to Paul Stavis, who served as counsel to three different New York State health agencies during his

---

[158] Id.

[159] Governor Cuomo, Statement of Disapproval for Senate Bill Number 3,184–A (September 23, 2011), available at: http://blog.nysarc.org/wp-content/uploads/2011/09/Veto-Message.jpg.

[160] Gale Scott, Calling Dr. Fraud, Crain's New York Business (March 21, 2010), available at: http://www.crainsnewyork.com/article/20100321/SUB/303219992.

[161] See supra note 153.

[162] See supra note 160.

[163] Comparison of Recoveries to date, NYS Global Cap report November 2012 compared to NYS Global Cap report November 2011, available at: http://www.health.ny.gov/health_care/medicaid/regulations/global_cap/monthly/docs/november_2012_report.pdf and http://www.health.ny.gov/health_care/medicaid/regulations/global_cap/monthly/docs/november_2011_report.pdf.

[164] Id.

28-   year health care career,[165] New York has made its Medicaid program "so utterly complicated that nobody completely under- stands it. It allows New York [S]tate to pull the wool over the feds' eyes." [166]

The Federal Government, particularly CMS, has been culpable in New York's historical Medicaid program integrity problems. No example better illustrates this failure better than CMS's approval of 35 modifications related to the excessive developmental center payment rate over the past 25 years. These modifications have collectively caused the State to receive an estimated $15 billion beyond a reasonable amount for just one, relatively small, part of the State's Medicaid program.

New York State has submitted several waiver applications to CMS that relate to the financing of its Medicaid program.[167] The Medicaid Redesign Team (MRT) Waiver Amendment asks CMS to allow New York to keep $10 billion of the anticipated Federal savings from the waiver. According to the State, it will use that money to increase primary care capacity, invest in new patient-centered models of care, strengthen safety-net programs and institutions, invest in the health care workforce, and improve management of chronic disease.[168]

Before considering the merits of these waivers, CMS and the State must come to an agreement to reduce the State's developmental centers to a rate of about one-fifth of their current levels, as CMS indicated was its intention at the September 20, 2012 hearing before the Subcommittee on Health Care, District of Columbia, Census and National Archives.

According to Dr. Feldman, "[w]hile Governor Cuomo has taken bold steps to redesign Medicaid in New York State, the Medicaid industrial complex is thriving, especially in New York City." [169] The Committee recommends six specific actions that should be taken immediately to reduce Medicaid waste, fraud, and abuse in New York's program and potentially save both Federal and New York State taxpayers significant amounts of money each year:

• CMS or a qualified government watchdog agency should conduct a complete and independent audit of New York's Medicaid program, including the work of New York State's Office of the Medicaid Inspector General;

• CMS should finalize an agreement with New York on a corrected payment methodology that ends the developmental center overpayments as soon as possible. CMS should pursue recovery of

---

[165] The complaints Mr. Stavis brought against New York's Medicaid program are discussed in Section III of this Report.

[166] Mary Beth Pfeiffer, Feds audit N.Y.'s Medicaid rates, Poughkeepsie Journal (May 14, 2011).

[167] See Achieving the Triple Aim, New York State Medicaid Redesign Team Waiver Amendment, New York State Department of Health, http://www.health.ny.gov/health_care/medicaid/redesign/docs/2012-08-06_waiver_amendment_request.pdf. See also It's Going to be a 1915 b/c Waiver, New York State Office for Persons With Developmental Disabilities, People First Waiver (June 6, 2012) available at http://www.opwdd.ny.gov/opwdd_services_supports/people_first_waiver/1915_b_c_waiver ("During discussions with CMS in May, OPWDD determined that a combination of a 1915 b and 1915 c waiver will provide the flexibility needed to redesign the delivery system to provide person-centered, need-focused supports and services as outlined under the People First Waiver. Therefore, OPWDD will pursue a combination of these two types of waivers rather than an 1115 Research and Demonstration Waiver.").

[168] New York State Medicaid Redesign Team (MRT) Waiver Amendment, available at: http://www.health.ny.gov/health_care/medicaid/redesign/docs/2012-08-06_waiver_amendment_request.pdf.

[169] See supra note 102.

an appropriate portion of previous overpayments in excess of reasonable costs for Federal taxpayers;
  • CMS' review of New York's Section 1115 waiver request to
allow the State to keep a portion of the savings its Medicaid reforms are projected to achieve, should follow all applicable statutory requirements, particularly with respect to budget neutrality.
CMS should also ensure that the baseline from which New York is
calculating the savings does not include developmental center overpayments or other overpayments;
  • New York's Personal Care Services program must only enroll
individuals who meet the eligibility thresholds required by law;
  • New York's legislature should ban "spousal refusal" and other
abuses of Medicaid eligibility rules, as Governor Cuomo has proposed in each of his three budgets. New York must also aggressively pursue estate recovery against people who abuse Medicaid
eligibility rules; and
  • New York's legislature should codify Governor Cuomo's executive order that limiting compensation of executives at organizations
receiving nearly all their money from tax revenue. New York must
also aggressively monitor and enforce these limits.

IX. CONCLUSION

In 2003, the Government Accountability Office (GAO) added
Medicaid to its list of high-risk programs.[170] This report highlighted significant problems in New York State's Medicaid program, and the previous section of this report outlined six specific
steps that CMS and New York can take to protect taxpayer dollars
from being misspent through New York's Medicaid program. Many
of the recommendations discussed in the report, such as limiting
Medicaid eligibility to individuals who meet the program's criteria,
limiting executive compensation at organizations that receive the
vast majority of their money through Medicaid, and strong state estate recovery programs should be implemented across the country.
  It is also important to note that CMS has struggled historically
in protecting Federal tax dollars from being misspent through Medicaid. CMS has been hampered by poor data quality, but the agency has historically failed to often adequately detect and address
major problems in state Medicaid programs. A Committee majority
staff report from April 2012 detailed several examples of how CMS
has failed to protect taxpayer dollars spent through the Medicaid
program.[171] Moreover, as GAO has widely reported, states have re-
sorted to creative techniques such as provider taxes and large supplemental payments to draw down additional Federal dollars into
their states through the Medicaid program without net State con-
tributions.[172] These techniques undermine the nature of joint Federal-state financial responsibility for the Medicaid program by significantly increasing the Federal share of Medicaid expenditures

---

[170] See Medicaid Waste, Fraud and Abuse, Threatening the Healthcare Safety Net: Hearing
Before the Senate Comm. on Finance, 109th Cong. (2005) (written statement of Kathryn G.
Allen, Health Care Director, Government Accountability Office), available at http://www.gao.gov/
new.items/d05836t.pdf.
[171] See supra note 1.
[172] U.S. Gov't Accountability Office (GAO): CMS Needs More Information on the Billions of
Dollars Spent on Supplemental Payments (2008), available at: http://www.gao.gov/new.items/
d08614.pdf.

and further undermining State incentives to run efficient Medicaid programs.

The national debt of the United States now exceeds $16.4 trillion, with more than $6 trillion added to the national debt in just the last four years. Congress faces critical and difficult choices about how to put the Federal budget on a sustainable path. The ideas in this report, which should receive bipartisan support, would alleviate some of the most egregious problems in the program and would begin to put the Medicaid program on a sustainable path.

APPENDIX A: PER CAPITA FEDERAL MEDICAID DOLLARS, BY STATE (FY2010)

State	Federal spending	State	Federal spending
New York	$1,655	Alabama	$769
Vermont	1,398	Texas	764
New Mexico	1,341	Oregon	761
Maine	1,295	Maryland	754
Louisiana	1,248	Iowa	742
Mississippi	1,184	Illinois	739
Rhode Island	1,170	Montana	737
West Virginia	1,143	New Jersey	716
Arizona	1,111	North Dakota	713
Massachusetts	1,107	Hawaii	705
Arkansas	1,095	Idaho	695
Alaska	1,056	California	695
Kentucky	1,033	Indiana	690
Tennessee	1,010	South Dakota	680
Missouri	1,008	Washington	659
Connecticut	990	Nebraska	650
Pennsylvania	972	Florida	624
Ohio	972	New Hampshire	623
South Carolina	888	Georgia	601
Delaware	885	Kansas	594
Minnesota	880	Wyoming	586
Michigan	865	Utah	499
North Carolina	855	Virginia	496
Oklahoma	841	Colorado	494
Wisconsin	809	Nevada	357

Medicaid expenditures by state as well as FMAP rates are from the Kaiser Family Foundation's state health care facts.[173] Population figures were obtained from the Census Bureau.

APPENDIX B: EXECUTIVE COMPENSATION AT NON-PROFITS FINANCED LARGELY BY MEDICAID

Organization	Position	2008 Compensation	2010 Compensation	County median household income
A C L D (Nassau Co)	Executive Director	$525,704	$552,761	$95,823
	CFAO	302,883	333,466	
	Assistant Executive Director	178,026	196,673	
	Assistant Executive Director	186,836	201,530	
Block Institute Inc (Brooklyn)	Executive Director/C E O	201,586	225,114	49,490
The Center for Discovery (Sullivan Co.)	C.E.O.	939,280	649,977	48,303
	Former C F O	480,832	N/A	
	C.F.O	254,595	238,293	
	Chief of Program	262,393	257,200	
	Chief of Admission	226,224	228,140	
	Chief of Health Services	248,725	223,398	

[173] Kaiser Family Foundation, Total Medicaid Spending, FY 2010, available at http://www.statehealthfacts.org/comparemaptable.jsp?ind=177&cat=4 (last visited January 3, 2012).

APPENDIX B: EXECUTIVE COMPENSATION AT NON-PROFITS FINANCED LARGELY BY MEDICAID—
Continued

Organization	Position	2008 Compensation	2010 Compensation	County median household income
	Chief of Development and Fundraising.	N/A	223,658	
Center for Disability Services Inc. (Albany Co.).	President/C E O	247,394	274,818	57,715
Community Services for the Developmentally Disabled (Buffalo).	President & C E O	*214,735	256,816	30,230
Developmental Disabilities Institute, Inc. (Suffolk Co)	Executive Director	294,576	N/A	87,187
	Associate Executive Director	225,589	280,356	
Epilepsy Foundation of Long Island (Nassau Co.).	Executive Director	*271,509	282,718	95,823
	C.F.O	175,174	214,502	95,823
Family Residences and Essential Enterprises Inc (Nassau Co.).	C.E.O	354,308	422,951	95,823
	C.F.O	218,146	285,323	
	Chief Compliance Office	234,193	251,422	
	Associate Director	175,271	201,718	
	Former C E O	858,587	N/A	
	C.O.O	N/A	261,327	
	Associate Director	N/A	215,714	
Federation Employment and Guidance Services (NYC).	C.E.O	533,323	582,513	51,270
	Executive Vice President	421,275	403,736	
	C.O.O	460,158	373,300	
	C.F.O	N/A	316,476	
	General Counsel	222,935	283,784	
	Chief Development Officer	N/A	267,569	
	Sr Vice President	271,870	292,378	
	Sr Vice President	256,144	277,437	
	Sr Vice President	204,587	227,979	
	Sr Vice President	260,302	276,405	
	Sr Vice President	206,998	221,836	
HASC Center Inc (Brooklyn)	Executive Director	*231,303	267,715	49,490
	Clinical Director	*244,929	259,641	
Head Injury Association Inc. (Suffolk Co.) ..	C.E.O	250,349	370,996	87,187
HeartShare Human Services of New York (Suffolk Co)	President and C E O	479,775	536,796	49,490
	Executive Vice President	317,449	318,481	
	Executive Director	231,284	247,020	
Human Care Services for Families & Children Inc (Brooklyn)	Executive Director	182,488	372,367	49,490
	C.F.O	132,603	234,894	
Independence Residences Inc. (Queens Co.)	Executive Director	232,213	267,190	56,406
	Associate Executive Director	177,627	206,171	
Institute for Community Living, Inc. (NYC)	C.E.O	752,330	3,048,520	51,270
	C.F.O	244,434	268,968	
	C.O.O	266,752	399,431	
	Sr. Executive Vice President	222,110	229,904	
	C.A.O	198,266	209,545	
	A.C.F.O	202,156	128,106	
Jawonio Inc (Rockland Co)	C.E.O	545,783	278,049	84,661
	Asst Exec Director	185,799	301,497	
Kelberman Center Inc (Oneida Co)	Treasurer/Secretary	*323,673	*334,139	48,382
Life's Worc Inc (Nassau Co)	Executive Director	378,502	395,828	95,823
	Assistant Executive Director of Operations.	182,092	209,280	95,823
LifeSpire Inc (NYC)	Unspecified	426,843	409,614	51,270
	Unspecified	209,651	222,119	
Maryhaven Center of Hope (Suffolk Co.)	C.E.O.	923,878	643,484	87,187
	Exec V P	778,990	1,003,980	
	C.F.O	344,459	429,328	
	V P Finance	231,698	244,565	

APPENDIX B: EXECUTIVE COMPENSATION AT NON-PROFITS FINANCED LARGELY BY MEDICAID—
Continued

Organization	Position	2008 Compensation	2010 Compensation	County median household income
NARCO Freedom Inc (Bronx)	C.E.O	382,690	386,018	41,057
NYSARC (Albany Co)	Executive Director	199,284	287,944	57,715
NYSARC (Chautauqua Co)	Executive Director/C E O	325,040	356,988	41,432
NYSARC (Madison/Cortland Co)	Executive Director	*214,635	237,848	53,473
NYSARC (Monroe Co)	C.E.O.	205,151	N/A	52,260
NYSARC (Montgomery Co)	C.E.O.	*1,630,083	512,420	43,254
NYSARC (Nassau Co)	C.E.O	*455,431	458,388	95,823
	Unspecified	*272,455	308,756	
	Unspecified	*285,394	348,077	
	Unspecified	*199,708	269,151	
NYSARC (NYC)	Assoc Executive Director	369,195	149,061	51,270
	Assoc Executive Director	327,896	422,456	
	Budget Director	300,300	371,766	
	Chief Compliance Officer	263,995	372,667	
	Senior Policy Advisor	243,661	666,444	
	Director of Employees	211,853	351,703	
NYSARC (Putnam Co)	Executive Director	*234,195	254,251	92,711
NYSARC (Suffolk Co)	C.E.O.	349,775	373,220	87,187
	Deputy Executive Director	197,470	215,494	
	Deputy Executive Director	198,699	224,673	
NYSARC (Sullivan Co)	C.E.O.	174,059	211,092	48,303
NYSARC (Westchester Co)	Executive Director	226,741	244,885	80,725
	Associate Executive Director	200,793	211,860	
Occupations Inc (Orange Co)	President/C E O	272,147	432,958	70,294
	Exec Vice President/ C O O	239,499	308,483	
	Vice President	119,875	304,884	
Ohel Childrens Home and Family Services (Brooklyn).	C.E.O	302,488	392,365	49,490
	C.F.O	227,906	248,510	
	Program Director	185,104	198,473	
	C.O.O	233,447	263,968	
	C.O.O	245,055	271,481	
	Chief Development Officer	297,179	319,405	
People Inc (Erie Co)	President/C E O	*424,640	472,419	48,805
	Vice President	*208,548	205,231	
Springbrook NY Inc (Ostego Co)	Executive Director	205,937	217,706	45,334
Staten Island Mental Health Society Inc. (Staten Island).	Unspecified	547,585	498,311	84,308
	Unspecified	190,249	209,342	
	Unspecified	233,740	208,732	
	Unspecified	209,513	223,753	
Westchester Institute for Human Development (Westchester Co)	President/C E O	*249,868	274,793	80,725
	C.O.O	*204,317	205,910	
Westchester School for Special Children (Westchester Co)	Executive Director	271,430	143,378	80,725
Young Adult institute (NYC)	President	2,106,905	954,912	51,270
	C.E.O.	1,991,753	1,089,518	
	Co-C O O	1,070,614	563,307	
	Co-C O O	1,191,809	605,039	
	CFO	404,220	432,339	
	Unspecified	242,973	N/A	
	Unspecified	292,927	319,309	
	Unspecified	221,903	264,948	
	Unspecified	257,510	276,322	
	Unspecified	238,650	288,440	
	Unspecified	N/A	330,755	

Notes Compensation amounts were found using publicly available IRS Form 990s accessed through guidestar
Denotes compensation for the year 2009 since 2008 data was not available through guidestar Median household income was obtained from Census Bureau County Quick Facts and is annual median household income for the period from 2007-2011 Median household income for Brooklyn, Staten Island, and the Bronx is from 2009 and was found at www city-data com

APPENDIX C: COMMITTEE'S METHODOLOGY FOR CALCULATING
MEDICAID OVERPAYMENTS

On July 19, 2012, the Committee sent a letter to Dr. Nirav Shah, Commissioner of the New York State Department of Health, asking for detailed information regarding overpayments received by New York State-operated developmental centers. Despite initial assurances from State officials that New York would respond to the Committee's request for information, the State decided not to comply. Because the State refused to comply with its request, the Committee compiled as much available information as possible from reliable sources in order to estimate the amount of overpayments received by New York State's developmental centers since 1990.

The Office of Inspector General (OIG) at the U.S. Department of Health and Human Services (HHS) supplied the Committee with a significant amount of information on these overpayments. Chiefly, OIG provided the actual payments received by New York developmental centers for state fiscal year (SFY) 2007 ($1.828 billion), SFY 2008 ($2.107 billion), and SFY 2009 ($2.267 billion), as well as the daily Medicaid payment rate per patient for New York's developmental centers over the entire period. Using the actual payments received by New York's developmental centers and OIG's calculations for reimbursable expenses, OIG estimated Medicaid overpaid the State developmental centers by $1.41 billion in SFY 2009, $1.359 billion in SFY 2008, and $1.063 billion in SFY 2007. The Committee requested that OIG estimate the developmental center overpayments over the past two decades using the same methodology it employed for its 2007–2009 estimates; however, OIG lacked the necessary information (the same information the State of New York has refused to provide the Committee) in order to perform the calculations.

It is important to note that OIG's calculation of overpayments relies upon the State's reported costs, and the State's reported costs were not verified or audited by either OIG or CMS. It is a complex formula with many supplementary and substantial add-ons that convert a prior year's reported costs into a current year's reimbursable costs. For example, New York's total reported costs for SFY 2008 were $581 million. After adding the various supplementary factors, OIG calculated the reimbursable cost for SFY 2009 was $858 million, about 48 percent higher than New York's reported costs for the previous year.

Therefore, there is reason to believe that the reimbursable costs calculated by OIG are significantly higher than are necessary to serve the State's developmental center population. According to the OIG report, the total reimbursement cost per patient was $1,532 per day for SFY 2009. Since OIG reported that the average rate received by similar, privately-operated Intermediate Care Facilities (ICFs) was $444 in SFY 2009, a $1,532 rate appears very high. Since OIG's report calculates overpayments by subtracting these inflated "reimbursable costs" from the payments received by State-operated developmental centers, the overpayments calculated by OIG for SFY 2007, SFY 2008, and SFY 2009 are likely substantially too low.

To avoid the shortcomings involved with OIG's somewhat nebulous "reimbursable costs," the Committee calculated the developmental center overpayments as the amount received by New York State-operated developmental centers in excess of the Medicaid Upper Payment Limit (UPL). According to Federal Medicaid law, the UPL is the maximum a given state Medicaid program can pay to Medicaid providers in the aggregate. To satisfy UPL requirements, Medicaid payments must not exceed what the Medicare program would pay for the same services. The Committee therefore estimated the Medicaid UPL using the most expensive Medicare payment category (see Footnote ii in the Table). Since the Committee's estimates used Medicare rates for the most costly patients in skilled nursing facilities (SNFs) and not all of the developmental center patients would fall into this category, the Committee's Medicaid UPL is almost certainly too high. Therefore, since the Committee is estimating the overpayments in excess of Medicaid UPL amounts and the Committee assumed the highest possible Medicare reimbursement rates, the Committee's estimates of the overpayments received by New York developmental centers are probably too low.

Medicare's reimbursement rates also vary by geographic location, and the State of New York has 14 geographic areas. The Committee calculated a weighted average of Medicare reimbursements using the geographic breakdown of the State's developmental centers in 2010. (This was the only year the Committee found an accounting of each developmental center's payment). Using developmental center population from that year, the Committee assigned Medicare payment regions the following weights: 37.19% to New York City, 21.10% to Binghamton, 15.81% to Rural New York State, 10.73% to Poughkeepsie, 8.75% to Rochester, 3.25% to Albany, and 3.18% to Buffalo. The Medicaid UPL estimates shown in the Table below for SFY 1999 through SFY 2011 were estimated using weighted average calculations. The Medicare payment information was easily obtainable only for the years after 1998. The average price change from 1999 to 2005 in Medicare's reimbursement rate for the most expensive patients in SNF was $12. Therefore, for purposes of the Committee's estimates, the Medicaid UPL was increased $12 each year from SFY 1991 to SFY 1998.

In order to calculate the estimated payments received by New York developmental centers, the Committee multiplied daily Medicaid payment rates per patient by the estimated number of patients residing in developmental centers at one point during the SFY. OIG provided the daily Medicaid payment rates and the Committee relied on reports issued by New York's Office for People with Developmental Disabilities (OPWDD) and its predecessor agency, the Office of Mental Retardation and Developmental Disabilities (OMRDD), to estimate patient numbers.[174] The fifth column in the Table shows the Committee's estimate of the amount Medicaid paid New York State-operated developmental centers beyond the Medicaid UPL (the amount Medicare would have otherwise paid). The second to last column is the present value of each year's estimated overpayment calculated using the consumer price

---

[174] OMRDD reports from 1999 to 2006 contained annual counts of the total residents in the State's developmental centers and OIG provided the actual reimbursements received by the State-operated developmental centers for 2007 through 2009. The sources for 1991, 1994, 2010, and 2011 are contained in the footnotes below the Table showing the estimated overpayments by year. For the remainder of the years (1992, 1993, 1995, 1996, 1997, and 1998), the Committee used a linear interpolation to estimate the number of developmental center residents.

index. Summing the overpayments from 1991 to 2011 yields a net estimated overpayment of nearly $28.8 billion beyond what was allowed by the Medicaid UPL. Finally, the last column shows the Federal share of the overpayments since the Federal Government reimburses at least half of New York's Medicaid expenditures. The total Federal overpayment (in present value terms) between 1991 and 2011 was approximately $15 billion.

TABLE—ESTIMATED MEDICAID OVERPAYMENT TO NEW YORK STATE-OPERATED DEVELOPMENTAL CENTERS

State fiscal year	Estimated dev. center patients	Daily dev center pay rate[i]	Estimated medicaid UPL[ii]	Over-payment	Overpayment present value (2011 $)[iii]	Federal share of overpayment [iv]
1991	[v] 6,350	$389	$319	[vi] $162.2M	$267.9M	$134.0M
1992	5,437	442	331	220.3M	353.2M	176.6M
1993	4,524	552	343	345.1M	537.2M	268.6M
1994	[vii] 3,611	654	355	394.1M	598.1M	299.1M
1995	3,294	936	367	684.2M	1,009.9M	504.9M
1996	2,978	1,093	379	776.0M	1,112.6M	556.3M
1997	2,661	1,310	391	892.7M	1,251.1M	625.5M
1998	2,345	1,522	403	957.6M	1,321.5M	660.8M
1999	[viii] 2,028	1,729	415	972.6M	1,313.2M	656.6M
2000	[ix] 2,020	1,930	426	1,108.9M	1,448.5M	724.3M
2001	[x] 1,711	2,165	435	1,080.4M	1,372.3M	686.1M
2002	[xi] 1,692	2,434	474	1,210.4M	1,513.7M	756.8M
2003	[xii] 1,599	2,723	457	1,322.5M	1,617.1M	808.6M
2004	[xiii] 1,610	2,934	483	1,440.3M	1,715.1M	882.9M
2005	[xiv] 1,696	3,063	490	1,592.8M	1,834.5M	944.4M
2006	[xv] 1,700	3,284	594	1,669.1M	1,862.4M	931.2M
2007	[xvi] X	3,715	613	1,526.3M	1,655.9M	827.9M
2008	[xvii] X	3,736	658	1,736.1M	1,813.8M	906.9M
2009	[xviii] X	4,116	645	1,911.4M	2,004.1M	1,090.0M
2010	[xix] 1,417	4,556	645	2,022.8M	2,086.6M	1,277.9M
2011	[xx] 1,313	5,118	751	2,092.9M	2,092.9M	1,274.3M
Total					28,781.6M	14,993.8M

[i] Development Center payment rates were according to the Office of Inspector General (OIG), Department of Health and Human Services

[ii] The Committee estimated the Medicaid UPL using the Medicare case-mix group with the highest reimbursement rate For FY 2006 to FY 2011, this group was the Rehabilitation Plus Extensive Services (RUX) group Beneficiaries classified under RUX generally have complex needs and require more assistance with activities of daily living, a greater amount of physical therapy, occupational therapy, and/or speech-language pathology services, and more complex clinical care For FY 1999 to FY 2005, the group with the highest reimbursement group was RUC from the Rehabilitation case-mix group Medicare s reimbursement rates also vary by geographic location and the State of New York has 14 geographic areas The Committee calculated a weighted average of the Medicare reimbursement using the geographic breakdown of the developmental centers in 2010 The following weights were assigned New York City 37 19%, Binghamton 21 10%, Rural New York State 15 81%, Poughkeepsie 10 73%, Rochester 8 75%, Albany 3 25%, Buffalo 3 18% Therefore the estimates in this category from FY 1999 to FY 2011 were estimated using weighted average calculations We used the average historical price change from 1999 to 2005 of $12 to estimate that Medicaid UPL increased $12 each year from FY 1991 to FY 1998

[iii] This column adjusts the overpayment column for 2011 values using the Consumer Price Index

[i] This calculation uses the State s Federal Medicaid Assistance Percentage (FMAP) Generally, New York s FMAP is 50% In fiscal years 2004, 2005, 2009, 2010, and 2011, the Federal Government increased the FMAP so the Federal share of the state s Medicaid expenditures in those years is higher New York s FMAP in SFY 2004 and SFY 2005 was 51 48% In SFY 2009, New York s FMAP was 54 39% In SFY 2010, New York s FMAP was 61 24% In SFY 2011, New York s FMAP was 60 89%

[v] Paul J Castellani, From Snake Pits to Cash Cows Politics and Public Institutions in New York, State University of New York, 2005, page 249

[vi] All of the figures in the table are in the millions This particular figure is $162 2 million

[vii] Castellani, supra note v, at 259

[ii] The 1998-99 Budget for the New York State Office of Mental Retardation and Developmental Disabilities

[ix] A Summary of the 1999-2000 Executive Budget Recommendation

[x] 2000-01 Executive Budget Recommendation for the New York State Office of Mental Retardation and Developmental Disabilities (OMRDD)

[xi] 2001-02 Fiscal Year Executive Budget Recommendations for OMRDD

[xii] 2002-03 Fiscal Year Executive Budget Recommendations for OMRDD

[xii] 2003-04 Fiscal Year Executive Budget Recommendations for OMRDD

[xi] 2004-05 Fiscal Year Executive Budget Recommendations for OMRDD

[xv] 2005-06 Fiscal Year Executive Budget Recommendations for OMRDD

[xvi] According to information provided by the OIG to the Committee, Medicaid made payments of $1,827,939,932 for State developmental centers in SFY 2007 Therefore, the Committee did not have to know the number of developmental center residents this year

[x] According to information provided by the OIG to the Committee, Medicaid made payments of $2,107,245,318 for State developmental centers in SFY 2007 Therefore, the Committee did not have to know the number of developmental center residents this year

[x iii] According to information provided by the OIG to the Committee, Medicaid made payments of $2,266,625,233 for State developmental centers in SFY 2007 Therefore, the Committee did not have to know the number of developmental center residents this year

[xix] Mary Beth Pfeiffer, At $4,556 A Day, N Y Disabled Care No 1 in Nation, POUGHKEEPSIE JOURNAL, June 20, 2010

[xx] OPWDD Statewide Comprehensive Plan 2011-2015

COMMITTEE CONSIDERATION

On February 14, 2013, the Committee met in open session and ordered reported favorably the report, Billions of Federal Tax Dollars Misspent on New York's Medicaid Program, as amended, by voice vote, a quorum being present.

STATEMENT OF OVERSIGHT FINDINGS AND RECOMMENDATIONS OF THE COMMITTEE

In compliance with clause 3(c)(1) of rule XIII and clause 2(b)(1) of rule X of the Rules of the House of Representatives, the Committee conducted oversight of the administration of Federal and state funds within New York's Medicaid program. The report includes findings from the Committee's investigation and recommendations to reduce waste, fraud, and abuse within the program.

STATEMENT OF GENERAL PERFORMANCE GOALS AND OBJECTIVES

In accordance with clause 3(c)(4) of rule XIII of the Rules of the House of Representatives, the Committee states that the report makes recommendations to stop Medicaid waste, fraud, and abuse in New York's Medicaid program, and potentially save both Federal and New York State taxpayers significant amounts of money each year.